Copyright © 2020 by Verona Jackson

RND

All rights reserved. No part of this publication may be reproduced, distributed, or transmitted in any form or by any means, including photocopying, recording, or other electronic or mechanical methods, without the prior written permission of the publisher, except in the case of brief quotations embodied in critical reviews and certain other noncommercial uses permitted by copyright law

Table of Contents

Introduction

The paleo diet, also known as the caveman diet, is one based off ancient eating practices. The diet avoids foods that our early ancestors wouldn't have been able to cook, like beans and grains, or foods that might have been unavailable, like milk or sugar. These easy foods follow those guidelines, and feature hearty cuts of meat along with a focus on fresh vegetables and fruit. Everything from salads to soups to skillet dinners are made paleo diet friendly in this collection of recipes.

Paleo Recipes to Try

Mushroom-Herb Chicken

Flavorful herbs and spices, red wine vinegar, shallots, and mushrooms give these plain chicken breasts rich flavor. A veggie side completes this paleo meal. If you don't care to use the red wine vinegar, you can use 1/3 cup of chicken broth.

Ingredients

- 4 (6-ounce) skinless, boneless chicken breast halves
- 1/4 teaspoon salt

- 1/4 teaspoon black pepper

- 1 teaspoon extra virgin olive oil, divided

- 3 large shallots, peeled (about 1 cup)

- 1 (8-ounce) package presliced mushrooms

- 1/3 cup red wine vinegar

- 1 teaspoon dried marjoram, crushed

- Freshly ground black pepper (optional)

Instructions

1. Place each chicken breast half between 2 sheets of heavy-duty plastic wrap; pound to 1/3-inch thickness using a meat mallet or small heavy skillet.

2. Sprinkle chicken evenly with salt and 1/4 teaspoon pepper and drizzle with 1/2 teaspoon olive oil. Heat a large nonstick skillet over medium-high heat.

3. Add chicken to pan, cook 5 to 6 minutes on each side or until browned.

4. While chicken cooks, cut shallots vertically into thin slices. Remove chicken from pan. Coat pan with 1/2 teaspoon olive oil.

5. Add mushrooms and shallots to pan. Cook 1 minute, stirring constantly. Stir in sherry and marjoram.

6. Return chicken to pan; cover and cook 3 to 4 minutes or until mushrooms are tender

and chicken is done. Transfer chicken to a platter.

7. Pour mushroom mixture over chicken; sprinkle with freshly ground pepper, if desired. Serve immediately.

Grilled Scallop Salad

Grill scallops and cucumber halves for tasty toppings on this fresh and flavorful salad. You'll love how the sweet watermelon and mint flavors play off one another. To make paleo-friendly, remove cooking spray.

Ingredients

- 1/2 teaspoon freshly ground black pepper, divided

- 3/8 teaspoon salt, divided

- 12 large sea scallops (about 1 1/2 pounds)

- 1 English cucumber, halved lengthwise

- Cooking spray

- 2 tablespoons fresh lime juice

- 2 teaspoons extra-virgin olive oil

- 4 cups torn romaine lettuce

- 3 cups (1-inch) cubed seedless watermelon

- 1/4 cup fresh mint leaves, torn

- 1/2 peeled avocado, cut into 8 slices

Instructions

1. Preheat grill to medium-high heat.

2. Sprinkle 1/4 teaspoon pepper and 1/4 teaspoon salt over scallops and cucumber. Arrange in a single layer on a grill rack coated with cooking spray.

3. Grill 3 minutes on each side or until scallops are done and cucumber is well marked.

4. Remove from heat; cut cucumber into 1/4-inch slices.

5. Combine remaining 1/8 teaspoon salt, juice, and oil in a large bowl; stir with a whisk.

6. Add cucumber, lettuce, watermelon, and mint; toss gently to coat. Divide the watermelon mixture evenly among 4 plates.

Top each serving with 3 scallops and 2 avocado slices.

7. Sprinkle evenly with remaining 1/4 teaspoon freshly ground black pepper.

8. **Sustainable Choice:** All scallops, whether farmed, diver-caught, or wild-caught, are great options.

Pork Chops with Fried Apples and Brussels Sprouts

Guaranteed to be a fast favorite, this recipe plays on the sweet-savory match made in flavor heaven:

pork + apples. Fried apples add a hint of sweetness and delightfully smooth texture to this hearty paleo pork dish. If you don't have access to Honeycrisp apples, use a pink lady, gala, or jazz apple instead.

Ingredients

- 12 ounces Brussels sprouts, halved
- 2 tablespoons extra-virgin olive oil, divided
- 5/8 teaspoon kosher salt, divided
- 1/2 teaspoon black pepper, divided
- 4 (4-ounce) boneless center-cut loin pork chops
- 2 tablespoons ghee, divided

- 12 ounces sliced Honeycrisp apple (1 large apple)

- 1/3 cup unsalted chicken stock

- 1/8 teaspoon ground nutmeg

- 3 tablespoons maple syrup

- 2 tablespoons Dijon mustard

- 1 tablespoon chopped fresh flat-leaf parsley

Instructions

1. Preheat broiler to high. Set the oven rack on the middle shelf.

2. Combine sprouts, 1 tablespoon olive oil, 1/4 teaspoon salt, and 1/4 teaspoon pepper in a bowl; toss to coat. Arrange sprouts in a

single layer on a jelly-roll pan coated with cooking spray. Broil 12 minutes, stirring every 3 minutes.

3. Heat a large skillet over medium-high heat. Add remaining 1 tablespoon olive oil; swirl to coat. S

4. prinkle pork with 1/4 teaspoon salt and remaining 1/4 teaspoon pepper; add to pan. Cook 3 minutes. Turn; cook 2 minutes or until done. Transfer pork to a plate.

5. Add 1 tablespoon ghee and apple to pan; fry 2 minutes.

6. Add stock and nutmeg; bring mixture to a boil. Stir in remaining 1/8 teaspoon salt, remaining 1 tablespoon ghee, syrup, Dijon

mustard, and parsley; cook 1 minute. Divide chops among 4 plates; top evenly with apple mixture. Serve with sprouts.

Paleo Skillet Chicken with Seared Avocados

One pan is all you need for this light and bright dinner. The tiniest bit of coconut sugar helps the avocado halves char in the pan, adding robust toasty flavor. While the original recipe called for sour cream, we kept it paleo by removing the drizzle.

Ingredients

- 1 tablespoon olive oil

- 4 (6-ounce) skinless, boneless chicken breast halves

- 1/2 teaspoon kosher salt, divided

- 1/2 teaspoon black pepper

- 1/2 teaspoon ground ancho chile powder

- 2 small ripe avocados, halved and pitted

- 1/4 teaspoon coconut sugar

- 2 medium red onions, peeled and cut into 1/4-inch-thick rings

- 4 green onions, trimmed

- 1 poblano pepper, sliced

- 3 tablespoons fresh lime juice

- 1 tablespoon Bragg liquid aminos

- 8 cilantro sprigs

- 4 lime wedges

- 1 teaspoon aleppo or other coarse red pepper (optional)

Instructions

1. Preheat oven to 450°.

2. Heat a large cast-iron skillet over medium-high heat.

3. Add oil to pan; swirl to coat. Sprinkle chicken with 1/4 teaspoon salt, black pepper, and chili powder.

4. Add chicken to pan; cook 4 minutes. Turn chicken over; cook 1 minute. Remove

chicken from pan (chicken will not be fully cooked).

5. Wipe pan clean with paper towels. Sprinkle avocados with coconut sugar.

6. Add avocados, cut side down, to pan; cook 2 minutes or until charred. Remove avocados from pan.

7. Add red onions; cook 3 minutes or until charred. Turn red onions; add green onions and poblano. Cook 3 minutes. Separate red onions into rings; toss with green onions and poblano.

8. Stir in lime juice and liquid aminos. Nestle chicken and avocados into onion mixture.

9. Place pan in oven; bake at 450° for 7 minutes or until chicken is done.

10. Remove pan from oven. Garnish with cilantro and lime wedges. Sprinkle with remaining 1/4 teaspoon salt and aleppo pepper, if desired.

Paleo Smoky Pork Tenderloin with Roasted Sweet Potatoes

Two teaspoons of smoked paprika may seem like a lot, but it will help to form a nice crust on the pork as it sears in the pan. You can also sub 1 teaspoon ground cumin plus 1 teaspoon chipotle chile powder. A hot oven will help the sweet potato wedges crisp up on the outside without burning.

Ingredients

- 1 (1-pound) pork tenderloin, trimmed
- 2 teaspoons smoked paprika
- 3/4 teaspoon kosher salt, divided
- 1/2 teaspoon freshly ground black pepper
- 1/2 teaspoon ground cumin
- 3 tablespoons extra virgin olive oil, divided
- 2 large sweet potatoes (about 11 ounces each), peeled and cut into 8 wedges each
- 1/4 cup cider vinegar

- 3 tablespoons maple syrup

- 1 teaspoon Dijon mustard

- 2 thyme sprigs

Instructions

1. Preheat oven to 450°.

2. Sprinkle pork evenly with paprika, 1/4 teaspoon salt, pepper, and cumin. Heat a large skillet over medium-high heat.

3. Add 1 tablespoon olive oil to pan; swirl to coat. Add pork to pan; cook 8 minutes, turning to brown on all sides.

4. Place potatoes on a baking sheet; drizzle with 1 tablespoon olive oil. Bake at 450° for 10 minutes.

5. Add pork to pan with potatoes; stir potatoes. Bake at 450° for 15 minutes or until potatoes are tender and a thermometer inserted into the thickest portion of the tenderloin registers 140°.

6. Remove pan from oven. Sprinkle potatoes with 3/8 teaspoon salt. Let pork stand 5 minutes before cutting into slices.

7. Combine remaining 1/8 teaspoon salt, vinegar, maple syrup, mustard, and thyme in a small saucepan; bring to a boil. Cook 3 minutes or until thickened.

8. Add remaining tablespoon olive oil, stirring with a whisk. Remove thyme sprigs; discard. Drizzle mustard mixture over potatoes. Serve with pork.

Chicken and Chile Hash

The mild flavor of spinach makes it wonderfully adaptable to sizzling garlic and spice from the crushed red pepper. For fullest flavor, cook spinach only until it begins to turn limp. Fried spinach can be made in a snap and pairs perfectly with almost every protein.

Ingredients

- 2 tablespoons water

- 12 ounces Yukon Gold potatoes, cubed

- 2 tablespoons olive oil, divided

- 1 teaspoon kosher salt, divided

- 1/4 teaspoon ground red pepper

- 12 ounces ground chicken

- 1 cup thinly vertically sliced red onion

- 1 poblano chile, seeded and chopped

- 2 cups cremini mushrooms, quartered (about 6 oz.)

- 1 tablespoon chopped fresh thyme, divided

- 5 garlic cloves, thinly sliced

- 3 tablespoons red wine vinegar, divided

- 4 large eggs

Instructions

1. Place 2 tablespoons water and potatoes in a microwave-safe dish; cover with plastic wrap. Microwave at High 5 minutes or until tender. Place potatoes on a paper towel-lined plate.

2. Heat a large cast-iron skillet over high. Add 1 tablespoon oil to pan; swirl to coat. Add 1/2 teaspoon salt, red pepper, and chicken; cook 5 minutes, stirring to crumble.

3. Remove chicken mixture to a bowl with a slotted spoon. Add onion and poblano chile to drippings in pan; cook 4 minutes. Add the mushrooms, 2 teaspoons thyme, and garlic;

cook 5 minutes. Add mushroom mixture to chicken mixture.

4. Add remaining 1 tablespoon oil to pan; swirl to coat. Add potatoes; cook 4 minutes, stirring occasionally.

5. Add remaining 1/2 teaspoon salt, chicken mixture, and 1 tablespoon vinegar to pan; cook 2 minutes.

6. Add water to a saucepan, filling two-thirds full; bring to a boil. Reduce heat; add remaining 2 tablespoons vinegar.

7. Break each egg into a custard cup, and pour each gently into pan; cook 3 minutes. Carefully remove eggs from pan using a slotted spoon.

8. Divide hash evenly among 4 plates; top with

    eggs and remaining 1 teaspoon thyme.

Paleo Sheet Pan Chicken with Roasted Baby Potatoes

A very hot oven quickly roasts the potatoes and finishes the chicken without overcooking. The simple oil mixture, using solely extra-virgin olive oil to keep it paleo-friendly, packs a ton of flavor without adding excessive calories or fat to an already flavorful dinner. To serve a family

Ingredients

- 8 ounces small Yukon gold potatoes (about 1 inch)
- 1 1/2 tablespoons plus 1 teaspoon extra-virgin olive oil, divided
- 1 tablespoon whole-grain mustard
- 1 tablespoon minced fresh tarragon
- 1 tablespoon apple cider vinegar
- 1 1/2 teaspoons minced fresh thyme
- 1 teaspoon honey
- 2 (6-ounce) skinless, boneless chicken breast halves
- 1/4 teaspoon kosher salt, divided
- 1/4 teaspoon freshly ground black pepper, divided

Instructions

1. Place a jelly-roll pan in oven. Preheat oven to 500° (leave pan in the oven as it preheats).

2. Carefully remove pan from oven. Add potatoes to pan; bake at 500° for 10 minutes.

3. Combine 1 1/2 tablespoons olive oil and next 5 ingredients (through honey) in a small bowl, stirring with a whisk.

4. Sprinkle chicken with 1/8 teaspoon salt and 1/8 teaspoon pepper. Heat a large skillet over medium-high heat.

5. Add 1 teaspoon olive oil to pan; swirl to coat. Add chicken to pan; cook 5 minutes. Turn

chicken over; drizzle chicken evenly with about 2 tablespoons mustard mixture.

6. Add chicken to jelly-roll pan with potatoes; bake at 500° for 10 minutes or until potatoes are tender and chicken is done.

7. Drizzle potatoes with remaining mustard mixture; sprinkle with remaining 1/8 teaspoon salt and remaining 1/8 teaspoon pepper.

Kale and Beet Salad with Salmon

White balsamic vinegar is slightly sweet; cider vinegar is tangier. Either will be delicious here. Canned salmon is an inexpensive, sustainable seafood option. Sub canned albacore tuna or 2 cooked salmon fillets.

Ingredients

- 2/3 cup plus 2 tablespoons cider vinegar, divided
- 1/2 cup water
- 1 tablespoon honey, divided
- 1 cup vertically sliced red onion
- 4 medium golden beets, trimmed

- 2 tablespoons olive oil

- 1 teaspoon Dijon mustard

- 1/4 teaspoon kosher salt

- 1/4 teaspoon black pepper

- 6 cups torn stemmed Lacinato or curly kale

- 2 (6-ounce) cans pink or red skinless, boneless salmon, drained and flaked (such as Wild Planet)

- 1/4 cup sliced almonds, toasted

Instructions

1. Bring 2/3 cup vinegar, 1/2 cup water, and 2 teaspoons honey to a boil in a small saucepan.

2. Add onion; boil 1 minute. Remove pan from heat, and let stand for 10 minutes. Drain.

3. Pierce beets a few times with a knife; wrap in a large piece of microwave-safe parchment paper. Microwave at High 7 minutes or until tender. Rub off skins with a paper towel. Halve beets; cut into wedges.

4. Combine remaining 2 tablespoons vinegar, remaining 1 teaspoon honey, oil, Dijon mustard, salt, and pepper in a large bowl.

5. Add beets and kale; toss to coat. Place about 1 1/2 cups kale mixture on each of 4 plates; top each with 3 ounces salmon, about 1/4 cup onion, and 1 tablespoon almonds.

Eggs in Purgatory

We're not entirely certain about the history of this classic recipe's name, but perhaps it has something to do with the spicy kick of the sauce. Our version is a shakshuka-like dish in which fiery harissa paste and heady spices slowly infused a rich tomato sauce where eggs gently poach.

Ingredients

- 1 tablespoon olive oil
- 1 cup chopped yellow onion (from 1 medium onion)
- 2 teaspoons ground cumin
- 1 teaspoon ground coriander

- 1 teaspoon smoked paprika

- 1/8 teaspoon ground cinnamon

- 4 garlic cloves, minced

- 1 (28-oz.) can unsalted crushed tomatoes

- 2 tablespoons harissa

- 3/4 teaspoon kosher salt, divided

- 8 large eggs

- 1 (5-oz.) pkg. baby spinach

- 1/4 cup chopped fresh cilantro

Instructions

1. Heat a large skillet over medium. Add oil to pan; swirl to coat. Add onion, and cook,

stirring occasionally, until translucent, about

4 minutes.

2. Add cumin, coriander, paprika, cinnamon,

and garlic; cook, stirring occasionally, until

garlic is soft and spices are fragrant, about

1 minute. Transfer to a 5- to 6-quart slow

cooker.

3. Stir in crushed tomatoes, harissa, and 1/2

teaspoon salt. Cover and cook on High 20

minutes; reduce heat to Low, and cook until

sauce is fragrant, 7 1/2 to 8 hours (or cook

on HIGH for 3 to 4 hours).

4. One at a time, crack eggs into a ramekin,

and slip into tomato sauce. (Do not stir.)

Cover and cook on HIGH until whites are set and yolks are runny, about 15 to 20 minutes.

5. Sprinkle eggs with remaining 1/4 teaspoon salt. Divide spinach evenly among 4 plates; top with sauce and eggs. Sprinkle with cilantro.

Slow Cooker Paleo Chicken, Bacon, and Potato Soup

This paleo soup is perfect for ushering in fall. It's hearty enough for the beginning of soup season, yet brothy and veggie-packed so that it doesn't feel too heavy. Pair it with a slaw or kale side salad for a light, satisfying dinner. This recipe is also ideal for a weekend.

Ingredients

- 4 center-cut bacon slices, diced
- 1 1/2 pounds bone-in chicken thighs, skinned
- 2 teaspoons salt-free garlic-and-herb seasoning blend (such as Mrs. Dash)
- 2 cups thinly sliced leek (from 2 large leeks)
- 1 cup sliced carrot (from 2 large carrots)
- 1 cup sliced celery (from 2 large stalks)
- 4 cups homemade chicken stock, divided

- 3/4 teaspoon kosher salt

- 1/2 teaspoon freshly ground black pepper

- 5 thyme sprigs

- 12 ounces sweet potatoes

- 2 cups coarsely chopped baby spinach

Instructions

1. Cook bacon in a large skillet over medium-high until crisp. Remove bacon from pan, reserving 1 teaspoon drippings in pan. Set bacon aside.

2. Sprinkle chicken with seasoning blend. Add chicken to bacon drippings in pan; cook 8 minutes, browning on all sides.

3. Transfer chicken using a slotted spoon to a 6-quart electric slow cooker, reserving any drippings in pan.

4. Add leek, carrot, and celery to drippings in pan; fry for 5 minutes. Stir in 1 cup stock, scraping pan to loosen browned bits.

5. Add leek mixture, bacon, remaining 3 cups stock, salt, pepper, and thyme sprigs to slow cooker. Cover and cook on LOW for 2 hours.

6. Add potatoes; cover and cook on LOW for 2 more hours or until potatoes are tender.

7. Remove chicken from slow cooker with a slotted spoon; discard thyme sprigs. Cut chicken into bite-size pieces; discard bones.

Return chicken to slow cooker; add spinach,

stirring until spinach wilts.

Pomegranate Curry Chicken

Talk about a company-worthy meal without much

effort or a hefty price tag. Serve this easy and

elegant entrée over a bed of greens and with a

side of steamed broccoli.

Ingredients

- 8 (3-oz.) skinless, boneless chicken thighs

- 1 teaspoon Madras curry powder

- 1/2 teaspoon kosher salt

- 1/2 teaspoon black pepper

- 1 1/2 teaspoons extra-virgin olive oil

- 1/4 cup pomegranate arils

- 2 teaspoons torn mint leaves

Instructions

1. Sprinkle chicken with curry powder, salt, and pepper. Heat oil in a large skillet over medium-high.

2. Add chicken to skillet; cook 5 minutes on each side or until done. Transfer chicken to a serving platter.

3. Sprinkle chicken with mint and pomegranate arils.

Burger Patty Salad

You can still enjoy all the taste of a juicy, veggie-topped burger without any of the excess calories due to a thick bun or heavy mayo-based sauce. This paleo salad features a hearty burger patty, fresh lettuce and tomatoes, and an herb-y vinaigrette to drizzle atop.

Ingredients

- 1/2 medium red onion

- 1/4 cup chopped parsley, divided

- 3/4 teaspoon black pepper, divided

- 5/8 teaspoon kosher salt, divided

- 1/4 teaspoon ground red pepper

- 1/4 teaspoon ground allspice

- 2 garlic cloves

- 6 ounces 90% lean ground beef

- 4 ounces lean ground lamb

- 1 large egg

- 2 tablespoons extra-virgin olive oil

- 1 tablespoon red wine vinegar

- 2 tablespoons fresh lime juice, divided

- 1 (5-oz.) pkg. baby kale leaves

- 1/2 English cucumber, thinly sliced

- 1 medium tomato, cut into 8 wedges

Instructions

1. Preheat broiler to high.

2. Cut onion half in half. Place 1 onion quarter in a food processor.

3. Add 2 tablespoons parsley, 1/2 teaspoon black pepper, 1/2 teaspoon salt, red pepper, allspice, and garlic; pulse until ground. Add beef, lamb, and egg; pulse to combine.

4. Shape beef mixture into 8 patties. Place patties on a jelly-roll pan; broil 6 minutes or until done.

5. Combine 1 tablespoon olive oil, red wine vinegar, 1 tablespoon lime juice, remaining 2 tablespoons parsley, 1/4 teaspoon black pepper, and 1/8 teaspoon salt.

6. Toss kale with remaining 1 tablespoon oil and 1 tablespoon lime juice. Slice remaining onion.

7. Divide kale mixture among 4 plates; top with sliced onion, sliced cucumber, and tomato.

8. Arrange 2 patties on each salad; drizzle evenly with vinaigrette.

Spicy Paleo Hash

Who knew a simple veggie dish could taste this flavorful? Cumin, cinnamon, and red pepper add warmth to this Peruvian-inspired sweet potato hash. For an added serving of protein, top it with a fried egg.

Ingredients

- 2 tablespoons olive oil
- 3 cups diced peeled sweet potato
- 2 tablespoons chopped fresh oregano
- 3/4 teaspoon kosher salt, divided
- 1/2 teaspoon ground cumin
- 1/2 teaspoon ground cinnamon

- 1/4 teaspoon ground red pepper

- 5 garlic cloves, minced

- 1 1/4 cups water, divided

- 1 cup green beans, trimmed and cut into 1-inch pieces

- 1/4 cup unsalted pumpkinseed kernels

- 1 plum tomato, seeded and diced

Instructions

1. Heat a large skillet over medium-high heat. Add oil to pan; swirl. Add potato, oregano, and 1/2 teaspoon salt; cook 3 minutes, stirring occasionally.

2. Add cumin, cinnamon, red pepper, and garlic; cook 1 minute. Add 1/2 cup water; cover, reduce heat, and cook 5 minutes. Uncover; cook 2 minutes. Remove pan from heat.

3. Bring remaining 3/4 cup water to a boil in a saucepan. Add remaining 1/4 teaspoon salt and green beans; cook 4 minutes.

4. Place 1/2 cup potato mixture in each of 4 shallow bowls; top each with 1 tablespoon pumpkinseeds and 1 tablespoon tomato.

Lamb Butternut Squash Stew

Tender lamb combines with fresh veggies like kale and butternut squash to create the ultimate comforting winter stew. Richly spiced with coriander, cumin, and paprika, the secret ingredient is also a dash of cinnamon. The best part of this simple paleo recipe is that the majority of the cooking time is hands-off, leaving you time to focus on other things.

Ingredients

- 8 ounces ground lamb
- 8 ounces 90% lean ground sirloin
- 1/2 teaspoon kosher salt, divided

- 1 1/2 cups chopped peeled butternut squash

- 1 cup chopped onion

- 2 garlic cloves, minced

- 1 tablespoon tomato paste

- 1/2 teaspoon ground coriander

- 1/2 teaspoon ground cumin

- 1/4 teaspoon ground paprika

- 1/4 teaspoon ground cinnamon

- 1 cup unsalted beef stock

- 3 cups chopped kale

- 2 tablespoons chopped fresh flat-leaf parsley

Instructions

1. Preheat oven to 450°.

2. Heat a large Dutch oven over medium-high heat. Add lamb, beef, and 1/4 teaspoon salt; cook 5 minutes or until browned, stirring to crumble.

3. Remove lamb mixture from pan. Add squash, onion, and garlic to pan; cook 3 minutes, stirring occasionally.

4. Add tomato paste and next 4 ingredients (through cinnamon); cook 1 minute, stirring frequently.

5. Stir in remaining 1/4 teaspoon salt and stock; bring to a boil. Stir in kale; cook 1 minute or until kale begins to wilt. Stir in

lamb mixture. Cover and bake at 450° for 15 minutes. Sprinkle with chopped parsley.

Dilly Salmon Packets with Carrots

Paleo meals don't have to be boring. Fresh dill and citrus add a pop of flavor to hearty salmon fillets and tender carrots. Remove the foil and arrange fillets over carrots for a lovely presentation.

Ingredients

- 4 (6-oz.) salmon fillets (about 1-in. thick)

- 4 tablespoons plus 1 teaspoon extra-virgin olive oil, divided

- 1/4 cup chopped fresh dill

- 1/2 teaspoon kosher salt

- 1/2 teaspoon black pepper

- 8 orange slices

- 1 pound small carrots, trimmed

Instructions

1. Preheat grill to medium-high heat.

2. Coat 4 (12-inch-square) pieces of foil each with 1/4 teaspoon olive oil; place 1 fillet in center of each piece. Top each fillet with 1 1/2 teaspoons olive oil and 1 tablespoon dill.

3. Top evenly with salt, pepper, and orange slices. Bring edges of foil up over fillets; fold to seal. Place packets, seal side up, on grill; cover and grill 12 minutes or until desired degree of doneness. Remove foil packets from grill.

4. Combine 2 tablespoons olive oil and carrots in a bowl; toss.

5. Place carrots on grill; grill 5 minutes or until crisp-tender, turning once after 3 minutes.

6. Divide carrots evenly among 4 plates. Open packets; top carrots with fillets. Squeeze orange slices evenly over fillets.

Mini Baked Sweet Potatoes

Mini spuds are a great gluten-free and paleo side for lighter mains like salads or soups. Look for small sweet potatoes about the size of your fist, or cook two larger potatoes and serve half a potato to each person.

Ingredients

- 4 (4-oz.) sweet potatoes
- 1 teaspoon extra-virgin olive oil
- 1/4 cup water
- 1/4 teaspoon kosher salt
- 4 teaspoons finely chopped chives

Instructions

1. Prick sweet potatoes liberally with a fork. Rub potatoes with oil. Place potatoes and 1/4 cup water in a microwave-safe baking dish; cover with plastic wrap.

2. Microwave at HIGH for 15 minutes or until tender, checking for doneness after 10 minutes. Cool slightly.

3. Partially split potatoes in half lengthwise; fluff flesh with a fork. Sprinkle with salt. Top evenly with chives.

Roasted Shrimp and Broccoli

Get dinner on the table quickly tonight by simply roasting shrimp and broccoli together for a quick, flavorful meal.

Ingredients

- 5 cups broccoli florets
- 1 tablespoon grated lemon rind, divided
- 1 tablespoon fresh lemon juice
- 1/2 teaspoon salt, divided
- 1/2 teaspoon freshly ground black pepper, divided
- 1 1/2 pounds peeled and deveined large shrimp

- Cooking spray

- 2 tablespoons extra-virgin olive oil

- 1/4 teaspoon crushed red pepper

Instructions

1. Preheat oven to 425°.

2. Cook broccoli in boiling water 1 minute. Drain and plunge into ice water; drain.

3. Combine 1 1/2 teaspoons rind, juice, 1/4 teaspoon salt, and 1/4 teaspoon black pepper in a medium bowl.

4. Add shrimp; toss to combine. Arrange broccoli and shrimp in a single layer on a jelly-roll pan coated with cooking spray.

Bake at 425° for 8 minutes or until shrimp are done.

5. Combine oil, remaining 1 1/2 teaspoons rind, remaining 1/4 teaspoon salt, remaining 1/4 teaspoon black pepper, and crushed red pepper in a large bowl.

6. Add broccoli; toss to combine.

Paleo Seared Scallops with Cauliflower Purée

Pair sea scallops with a cauliflower and potato purée for an elegant yet weeknight-friendly meal.

Ingredients

- 2 cups chopped cauliflower florets

- 1 cup cubed peeled Yukon gold potato

- 1 cup water

- 1/2 cup all-natural chicken broth

- 1 tablespoon extra-virgin olive oil

- 1 1/2 pounds sea scallops

- 3/4 teaspoon kosher salt, divided

- 1/2 teaspoon coarsely ground black pepper

- 1 1/2 tablespoons ghee

- 1/8 teaspoon crushed red pepper

Instructions

1. Bring first 4 ingredients to a boil in a saucepan; cover, reduce heat, and simmer 6 minutes or until potato is tender.

2. Remove from heat. Let stand, uncovered, 10 minutes.

3. Heat a large skillet over high heat. Add olive oil; swirl to coat. Pat scallops dry with paper towels; sprinkle with 1/4 teaspoon salt and black pepper.

4. Add scallops to pan; cook 3 minutes on each side or until desired degree of doneness. Remove scallops from pan.

5. Pour cauliflower mixture in a blender. Add 1/2 teaspoon salt, ghee, and red pepper.

6. Remove center piece of blender lid (to allow steam to escape); secure lid on blender.

7. Place a clean towel over opening in lid (to avoid splatters). Blend until smooth. Serve puree with scallops.

Shrimp Cauliflower Fried Rice

This flavorful paleo bowl is an easy and healthy way to liven up your next dinner. Topped with hearty shrimp and loaded with aromatic fresh ginger, this is a special meal that the entire family can get excited about.

Ingredients

- 1/2 pound peeled and deveined shrimp

- 1 teaspoon grated peeled fresh ginger

- 1/4 teaspoon crushed red pepper

- 2 teaspoons dark sesame oil

- 1/3 cup chopped red bell pepper

- 1/2 cup sliced green onions

- 1 tablespoon bottled minced garlic

- 4 cups riced cauliflower

- 1 large egg, lightly beaten

- 2 tablespoons liquid aminos

- 1 tablespoon water

Instructions

1. Combine shrimp, ginger, and crushed red pepper in a small bowl; let stand 5 minutes.

2. Heat oil in a large nonstick skillet over high heat. Add bell pepper, green onions, and garlic; stir-fry 1 to 2 minutes or until tender.

3. Add shrimp mixture to pan; stir-fry 4 to 5 minutes or until shrimp are done.

4. Add riced cauliflower; stir-fry 2 minutes or until thoroughly heated. Push rice mixture to sides of pan, forming a well in center.

5. Add egg to center of pan, and cook 30 seconds; toss with rice mixture, and stir-fry until egg is cooked.

6. Stir in liquid aminos and water; cook until thoroughly heated.

Spiralized Puttanesca

Spiralized sweet potatoes make for a hearty pasta replacement in this fresh feeling paleo meal. Puttanesca is an ultra-savory Italian pasta dish that typically consists of capers, anchovies, olives, tomatoes, garlic, and olive oil. For a vegetarian option, leave out the anchovies and use vegetable broth instead of chicken.

Ingredients

- 1/4 cup extra-virgin olive oil

- 6 garlic cloves, minced

- 4 anchovy fillets

- 1 1/2 teaspoons dried oregano

- 3/4 teaspoon crushed red pepper

- 2 cups unsalted chicken stock

- 6 cups spiralized sweet potatoes

- 3 pints multicolored cherry or grape tomatoes, halved

- 2 tablespoons unsalted tomato paste

- 1/4 cup chopped fresh basil

- 1/4 cup chopped fresh parsley

- 24 pitted kalamata olives, chopped

- 3 tablespoons capers

- 1/8 teaspoon salt

Instructions

1. Heat a large high-sided fry pan over medium heat.

2. Add oil to pan; swirl to coat. Add garlic, anchovies, oregano, and red pepper; cook 2 minutes, stirring constantly to break up anchovies.

3. Add stock and bring to a boil. Stir in spiralized sweet potatoes, tomatoes, and tomato paste. Cook 2 to 3 minutes or until the sweet potatoes have slightly softened.

4. Remove pan from heat; add remaining ingredients, tossing to combine.

Blackened Steak Salad

Steak-centric salads are a staple of the American gastropub menu. Unfortunately, the salad interpretation is a bit loose—the lettuce merely a bed for a Flinstone-sized protein serving, the butter-yellow croutons, tons of cheese, and creamy dressing blanketing all.

Ingredients

- 1/2 teaspoon kosher salt

- 1/2 teaspoon black pepper

- 1/2 teaspoon paprika

- 1/4 teaspoon garlic powder

- 1 (12 oz.) flank steak, trimmed

- 1/4 cup extra-virgin olive oil

- 2 tablespoons balsamic vinegar

- 1 teaspoon Dijon mustard

- 4 cups firmly packed arugula

- 1/2 cup vertically sliced red onion (from 1 small onion)

- 1/2 ripe avocado, chopped

Instructions

1. Heat a grill pan over medium-high. Combine salt, pepper, paprika, and garlic powder in a small bowl. Rub spice mixture evenly over steak.

2. Add steak to pan; grill 5 minutes on each side for medium-rare or until desired degree of doneness.

3. Place steak on a cutting board. Let stand 5 minutes. Cut across the grain into thin slices.

4. Combine oil, vinegar, and mustard in a large bowl, stirring with a whisk.

5. Add steak, arugula, and onion; toss to coat. Divide salad among 4 plates. Top evenly with avocado.

Skillet Chicken with Escarole and Pecorino

Escarole is amped up with a salty kick from fish sauce and is brightened with sweet, crunchy carrots. To make paleo-friendly, omit pecorino cheese.

Ingredients

- 1 pound escarole, cut into wide ribbons

- 2 tablespoons plus 2 teaspoons extra-virgin olive oil, divided

- 4 (4-ounce) chicken breast cutlets

- 3/8 teaspoon kosher salt

- 1/4 teaspoon freshly ground black pepper

- 4 large garlic cloves, crushed

- 1/4 teaspoon crushed red pepper

- 1/2 medium red onion, thinly sliced

- 2 teaspoons fish sauce

- 1/4 cup julienne-cut carrot

- 1/2 ounce pecorino Romano cheese, shaved

Instructions

1. Bring a saucepan of water to a boil over high heat. Add escarole; cook 1 minute. Drain.

2. Heat 2 teaspoons oil in a skillet over medium-high heat. Sprinkle chicken evenly with salt and pepper.

3. Add chicken; cook 2 minutes on each side or until done. Transfer to a plate.

4. Reduce heat. Add remaining 2 tablespoons oil and garlic; cook 1 minute. Stir in red pepper and onion; cook 1 minute.

5. Remove garlic from pan; discard. Add escarole; cook 1 minute. Stir in fish sauce.

6. Divide chicken among 4 plates; top with escarole, carrot, and cheese.

Creamy Sweet Potato Soup

Microwaving, instead of roasting, the sweet potatoes saves more than an hour. To make paleo-friendly, omit the Parmesan cheese.

Ingredients

- 2 pounds sweet potatoes, halved lengthwise (about 2 large)
- 1/4 cup water
- 2 teaspoons olive oil
- 1 cup chopped onion
- 1/2 teaspoon ground cumin
- 1/4 teaspoon crushed red pepper

- 4 cups unsalted chicken stock (such as Swanson)

- 1/4 teaspoon salt

- 6 bacon slices, cooked and crumbled

- 1 ounce fresh Parmesan cheese, shaved (about 1/4 cup)

- 2 tablespoons flat-leaf parsley leaves (optional)

Instructions

1. Place potatoes, cut sides down, in an 11 x 7-inch microwave-safe baking dish.

2. Add 1/4 cup water; cover with plastic wrap. Microwave at HIGH 15 minutes or until

potatoes are tender. Cool slightly; discard potato skins.

3. Heat a saucepan over medium-high heat. Add oil; swirl to coat. Add onion; fry for 1 minute or until translucent. Stir in cumin and red pepper.

4. Add stock to pan; bring to a boil. Place half of sweet potato and half of stock mixture in a blender.

5. Remove center piece of blender lid (to allow steam to escape); secure blender lid on blender.

6. Place a clean towel over opening in blender lid (to avoid splatters); blend until smooth. Pour pureed soup into a large bowl. Repeat

procedure with remaining sweet potato and stock mixture. Stir in salt.

7. Divide soup evenly among 6 bowls; sprinkle cooked bacon and Parmesan cheese evenly over top. Garnish with parsley, if desired.

Beef and Broccoli Stuffed Sweet Potatoes

Russets aren't the only spuds worth stuffing. Smoke and heat, achieved with chili powder and ground red pepper, work particularly well with sweet potatoes. This makes for a great paleo main dish, or cut them smaller and serve open-faced as a Super Bowl-style appetizer.

Ingredients

- 4 (8-oz.) sweet potatoes
- 1 tablespoon extra-virgin olive oil, divided
- 1 cup chopped red onion
- 3/4 cup drained and chopped bottled roasted red bell peppers
- 4 garlic cloves, minced
- 2 teaspoons chili powder
- 1/2 teaspoon kosher salt, divided

- 1/2 teaspoon ground cumin

- 1/4 teaspoon ground red pepper

- 10 ounces 90% lean ground sirloin

- 2 cups frozen steam-in-bag broccoli florets

- 1/4 cup chopped green onions

Instructions

1. Rub sweet potatoes with 1 1/2 teaspoons oil; pierce several times with a fork. Microwave at HIGH 12 to 15 minutes or until potatoes are tender.

2. Heat a large skillet over medium-high. Add remaining 1 1/2 teaspoons oil; swirl to coat.

3. Add onion and red bell peppers; cook 5 minutes or until tender, stirring frequently.

4. Add garlic, and cook 3 minutes, stirring frequently. Stir in chili powder, 1/4 tea¬spoon salt, cumin, and ground red pepper.

5. Add beef; cook 6 minutes or until browned, stirring to crumble.

6. Heat broccoli according to package directions; stir into beef mixture. Partially split potatoes lengthwise; fluff the flesh with a fork. Top potatoes evenly with beef mixture, remaining 1/4 teaspoon salt, and green onions.

Honey and Sesame-Glazed Chicken Breasts with Green Beans

Sweet honey and toasty sesame team up for a flavor combo everyone at the table is sure to love. To make paleo-friendly, substitute ghee for butter.

Ingredients

- 6 tablespoons unsalted chicken stock

- 1/3 cup honey

- 2 tablespoons dark sesame oil, divided

- 1 1/2 tablespoons whole-grain mustard

- 4 (6-ounce) skinless, boneless chicken breast halves

- 3/4 teaspoon kosher salt, divided

- 1/2 teaspoon freshly ground black pepper, divided

- 2 teaspoons toasted sesame seeds

- 2 (8-ounce) packages trimmed fresh green beans

- 1 tablespoon unsalted butter, melted

- 2 tablespoons sliced almonds, toasted

Instructions

1. Combine chicken stock, honey, 1 tablespoon oil, and mustard in a small saucepan over medium-high heat, stirring with a whisk; bring to a boil.

2. Reduce heat; cook 10 minutes or until syrupy, stirring occasionally.

3. Heat a large nonstick skillet over medium-high heat.

4. Add remaining 1 tablespoon oil to pan; swirl to coat. Sprinkle chicken with 1/2 teaspoon salt and 1/4 teaspoon pepper.

5. Add chicken to pan; cook 6 minutes on each side or until done. Pour honey mixture over chicken, and sprinkle with sesame seeds.

6. Prepare green beans according to package directions. Combine remaining 1/4 teaspoon salt, remaining 1/4 teaspoon pepper, butter, and beans in a bowl; toss to coat. Sprinkle with almonds.

Paleo Spaghetti Squash Shakshuka

Shakshuka, a traditional Israeli breakfast food, is a skillet of spiced tomatoes, peppers, and onions with baked eggs. In this version, we swapped out our trusted cast-iron skillet for the walls of a spaghetti squash boat to create a paleo-friendly morning meal.

Ingredients

- 1 medium spaghetti squash
- 2 tablespoons extra virgin olive oil
- 1/2 medium yellow onion, chopped
- 1 large garlic clove, minced
- 1 red pepper, chopped

- 1 jalapeño, seeded and chopped

- 1 (15-oz.) can diced, unsalted tomatoes

- 1 teaspoon cumin

- 3/4 teaspoon chili powder

- 1/2 teaspoon kosher salt

- 2 large eggs

- 2 tablespoons finely chopped fresh cilantro

Instructions

1. Preheat oven for 425°F. Using a fork, poke the spaghetti squash several times all over.

2. Microwave for 10 minutes on high, flipping half way through the cook time.

3. Cut squash in half and remove seeds. Using a fork, gently scrape the flesh to form spaghetti strands.

4. In a medium skillet over medium heat, add oil, onion, and peppers. Cook until slightly softened, about 5 minutes.

5. Add garlic. Fry 1 minute. Add canned tomatoes, cumin, chili powder, salt, and pepper, and let simmer 10 minutes.

6. To construct the dish, divide the sauce among each of 4 squash halves.

7. Using a spoon or spatula, fully mix the tomato sauce with squash strands. Make a divot in the center of each boat and crack an egg into the divot.

8. Place each squash half on a baking sheet. Use aluminum foil to secure the squash halves if they roll. Bake 10 minutes.

9. Remove from oven, top with cilantro, and serve immediately.